EMOTIONS VERSUS HEALTH
IN WOMEN

BY

MARY T. BISSELL, M. D.

ISBN-13:
978-1727077780

ISBN-10:
1727077784

WHEN the harassed and wretched Macbeth inquired of the doctor, "Canst thou not minister to a mind diseased?" his candid physician promptly disclaimed any such high qualifications. "Therein," said he, "the patient must minister to himself."

It is possible that the modern physician would appear less modest under a similar interrogation, since modern hygiene claims the entire man for its operations, concerning itself not only with his physical, but also with his mental good. Keenly alive to the intimate relations existing between mind and body, it often throws upon the physician of to-day the responsibility of determining whether the remedy indicated be chemical or spiritual. This broad outlook embraces large and small interests, and may certainly include one feature in the training of women which, we believe, is opposed to her best growth and health. We refer to a tendency which exists in her education to an undue stimulation of her emotional nature.

Woman is believed to have been endowed by Nature with a strongly emotional temperament. She is accepted as the fairest exponent of sentiments, which in turn lend her her chiefest charm. Tears and smiles, emotion and sensibility, are expected of her. It is permitted to her to be a blue-stocking if she will, but sympathetic and tender she must be. If Hypatia has her admirers, all the world loves Juliet! It is precisely in that natural aptitude for emotion, in that type of mind which is exquisitely sensitive to impressions and generously swayed by sympathetic feeling, that one of the great dangers to the perfection of womanhood, physical and mental, may be said to reside.

Many and varied influences tend to increase this emotional excitability until it often becomes a fixed habit of mind; an undue sensibility of the supreme centers to emotional ideas is created, which can only be maintained at the expense of sound health of body and of mind. First among these are certain home influences that are brought to bear upon a little girl from her earliest childhood, which foster in her self-consciousness and introspection.

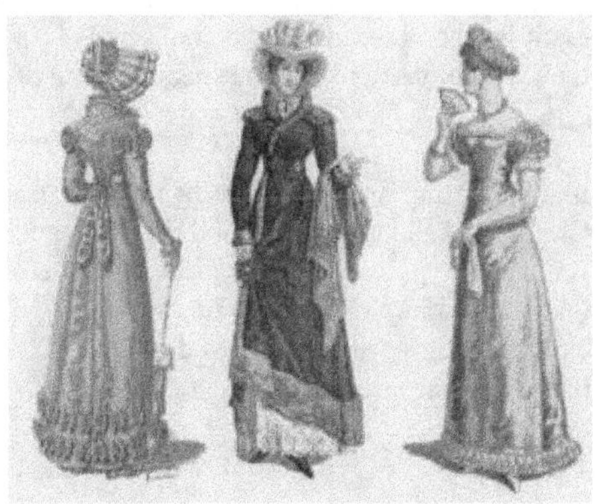

She is generally permitted narrower limits,
within which she can play, can dress, can
succeed, than are allowed to her brother,
even when her physique is equally able. She
is housed more closely, her out-of-door
sports are fewer and less interesting, and her
dress is too often a limitation to her
freedom. Such restrictions of her liberty, and
constant reference to the fact that her sex
denies her this or that employment or
pleasure, tend to make a child self-conscious
and emotionally overactive. Methods of
family discipline which depend upon
appeals to the emotional natures of children
have like unhealthy results, for they promote
a condition of mental commotion and unrest
harmful to children, who require an even
atmosphere for the mind as well as for the
body. There are often undue claims made
upon little children for the demonstration of
their affections, and this is especially true of
girls.

In a paper on "Emotional Prodigality among
Children," read before a dental society some
years ago by Dr. C. F. Taylor, it was argued
that stimulation of the emotions among
children conduced not only to diseases of
the spine, but also to dental caries.

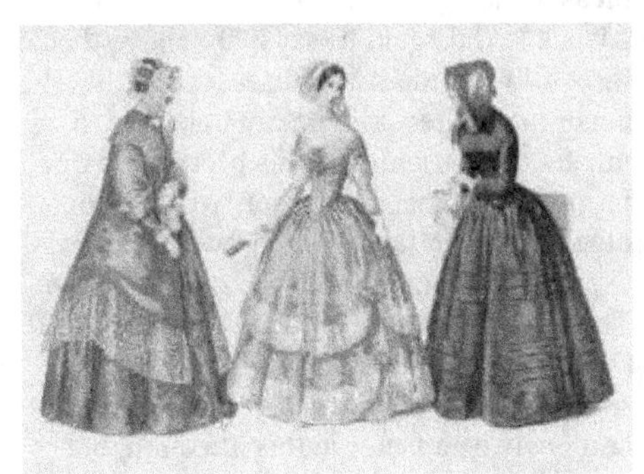

Dr. Taylor says: "In my large practice among children, I am certain that scores are literally killed by the excessive amount of emotional excitement which they are forced to endure. All this hugging and kissing and talking to them is to excite responses of the same emotional nature in the child for the pleasure and gratification of the parents and friends." And again he says: "I believe that three fifths of the spinal diseases which occur in children are directly traceable to mental overaction. And this because a large proportion of these cases gets well without other treatment than a withdrawal from the exciting cause of emotional disturbance." The writer does not subscribe to this view of the causation of lateral curvature, except in so far as any influence which weakens the body may be a factor in this affection, but the opinion is of interest as suggesting the extent of this and kindred influences.

The literature which little girls are permitted to read may be held responsible for much emotional stimulation of an unhealthy character. If a man be known by the company he keeps, it is equally true that he is known by the books he reads. The last quarter of a century has opened a wide vista of healthful delight for children through the green fields of modern child literature, but the prospect is not yet entirely fair. The hot-house atmosphere prevails in many volumes, which owe their birth to the present decade.

I recall a very popular series of girls' books, widely read at the present time, in which the emotional natures of the little heroines are continually maintained at concert pitch from the strain put upon them by appeals to affection, to conscience, to inordinate love of praise, etc. I have often been astonished to see intellectually promising and otherwise sensible little girls devouring pages of unhealthy sentiment such as would fill their robust little brothers with scorn and repugnance.

We need only briefly refer to the unhealthy influence exerted upon the minds of little girls by foolish indulgence in showy dress or in social dissipation. Dissipation, indeed, is a serious term to apply to the social pleasures of little children, but, when we hear of children's parties beginning at nine o'clock, in which toilets and manners only suitable for their mammas are encouraged, we easily conclude that, in the lack of simplicity in social customs, we may find an abnormal stimulus to the emotional natures of American girls.

Certain school influences have a large responsibility in this direction. What is called the hot-house pressure of public schools, and the elaborate system of examinations in our higher institutions of learning, have their evil not in the exercise of the calmer faculties of the mind, such as judgment, reason, memory, etc., but in their tendency to arouse that complex emotion called *worry*. These influences are exerted, it is true, upon girls and boys alike, but, as the facility of the girls for emotional disturbance is greater, they suffer more largely per consequence. The repeated stimulation of such complex emotions can not fail to agitate the mind of young girls, and insidiously disturb its calm.

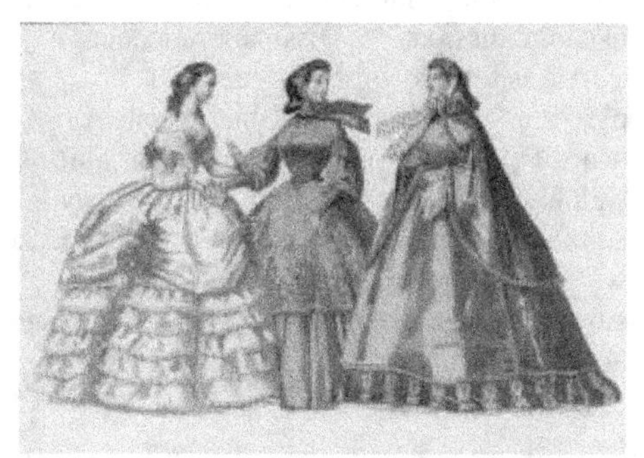

As the girl grows to womanhood, the
impression made by these influences upon
her plastic child nature can not be entirely
thrown off. If she be of a strong and
womanly type, she will meet the physical
and social trials of life with such character
and self-possession as she may, but they will
have for such a one a double force. Life
offers only too many facilities for overtaxing
the sympathies of the unduly sensitized
individual. The appeals of misery, poverty,
and sorrow sound in every ear. The woman
who would maintain a just equilibrium
between sentimental mourning and efficient
sympathy for these facts of existence needs
to be re-enforced, not weakened, by the
education of her childhood. And if to the
friction of any life we add the strain of an
elaborate social system, if our young woman
be a society girl, with all the demands of a
high-bred life of fashion upon her time,
temper, versatility, and self-control, we have
one more influence which maintains her at
constantly high emotional pressure.

It is evident that the sum of these and similar
forces constantly exerted upon the mind of
women must have their due effect. The
normal result of the stimulation of any organ
of the body is well known to be a final loss
of health in that organ. When the faculties of
the mind, called out in the display of the
emotions, are overtaxed. we generally find
either a lack of will-power or a deficiency in
reason and judgment, and our common
expression for that condition is that such an
individual is not well balanced.

It is possible that some of us have heard it
suggested that woman is a less reasonable
being than man. It has, indeed, been

whispered that she—regarding her as a type, not as an individual—is less logical, less temperate in her judgments, more easily controlled by appeals to the feelings. In the recent article by Ouida in the "North American Review," speaking of the character of a woman's mind, she says: "The female mind has a radical weakness, which is often also its peculiar charm; it is intensely subjective; it is only reluctantly forced to be impersonal." Such opinions are not entirely unfamiliar to any of us.

We are in no wise concerned for the final judgment of mankind upon the mind of woman, nor do we imagine that it requires championship. But it is easily apparent that this very grace of her nature may be turned to bad account through undue stimulation, and that, through inheritance and the influences we have briefly suggested, she may acquire a tendency toward an unduly subjective type of mind—a tendency which threatens the loss of a just intellectual sense of proportion, and which, therefore, can not conduce to sound mentality.

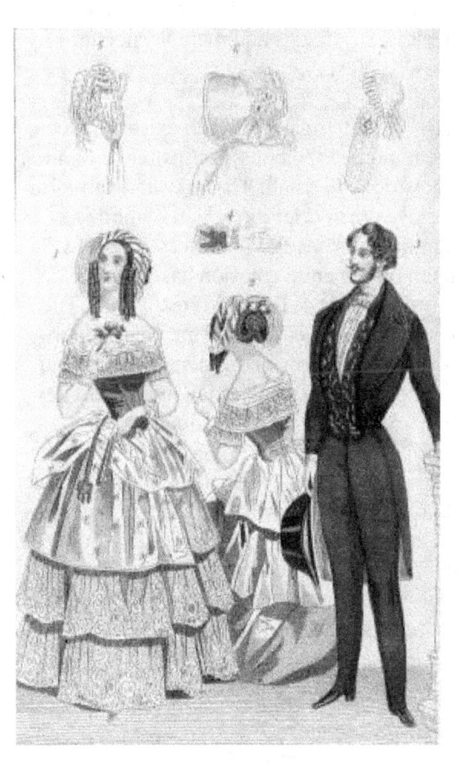

The old meaning of the word emotion—*commotion*—is opposed to the best mental growth and health. In repose, in the quiet harmonious performance of its functions, the mind grows into vigorous maturity, and the constant unrest and commotion of nerve-elements, which accompany violent emotional disturbances, and repeated strain upon other than its reasoning faculties, can not fail to disturb the quiet, natural evolution of its powers. Can this tendency in woman's training be shown to affect her bodily health? Physicians and metaphysicians answer. Yes!

The intimate relation which exists between the mind and the body is a matter of familiar knowledge to us all. The tear that starts from the eye when grief disturbs the mind is a common instance of the effect which an intangible mental emotion has upon the physical basis of the lachrymal gland. The loss of consciousness and the heart-failure which may follow great mental shock, and the deleterious effect which mental anxiety may exercise upon digestion, are, unfortunately, matters of common experience. Even the poetical allusion to the hair which grows white in a single night has its basis in physiological fact. The miracles claimed by the faith-curers are in the same Hue of argument, for they indicate how far sedation of the mind may be an adjuvant to the cure of the body.

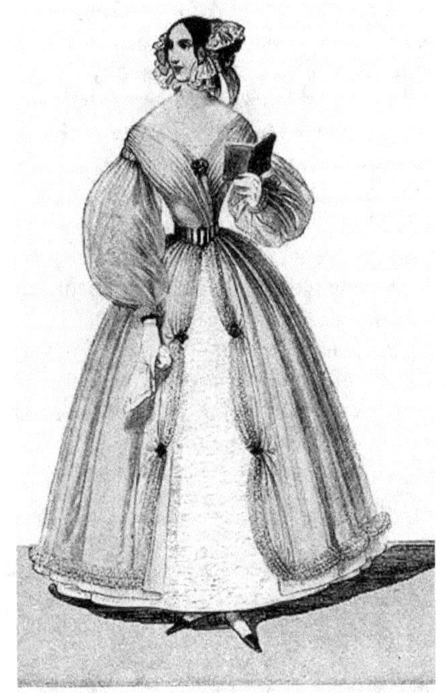

" WIENER ZEITSCHRIFT."   March 1840

Says Maudsley: "It may be questioned whether there is a single act of nutrition which emotion may not affect, infecting it with feebleness, inspiring it with energy, and so aiding or hindering recovery from disease. It is certain that joy or hope exerts an animating effect upon the bodily life, quiet and equable when moderate, but when stronger, evinced in the brilliancy of the eye, in the quickened pulse, in an inclination to laugh and sing; grief, or other depressing passion has an opposite effect, relaxing the arteries, enfeebling the heart, making the eye dull, impeding digestion, and producing an inclination to sigh or weep." This exaggeration of the emotions, seen in many cases among women, may be considered a serious factor in inducing some of the most common diseases of the nervous system from which Americans, in particular, are suffering.

In his treatise on the causes of these nervous diseases Dr. Ross, of London, says: "Psychical disturbances are a prolific source of disease of the nervous system, and it is probable that as civilization advances these causes will exercise a more and more predominant influence in the production of nervous disease. The depressing passions, such as fright, alarm, disgust, terror, and rage, have, no doubt, in all ages, exerted a deleterious influence on the nervous system; but in the present day the keen competition evoked by the struggle for existence in the higher departments of social life must subject the latest evolved portion of the nervous system to a strain so great, that those only possessing the strongest and best balanced nervous system can escape unscathed." Of these nervous diseases,

nervous exhaustion and hysteria were never
more rife than to-day.

As regards the occurrence of hysteria, while
it is frequently found among those belonging
to what we call the lower classes of society,
it is more frequently manifested among the
more highly cultivated. A French author
who, indeed, speaks for his own country
only, states that one out of four of all
females are decidedly affected with hysteria,
and that one-half present an undue
impressionability which differs very little
from it. Although these statistics are too
high for America, they are significant as
being possible anywhere, and not the less so
as coming from a land where, if a woman is
anything, she is emotional.

Among the frequent causes of hysteria, all
writers mention the depressing passions,
such as fear, anxiety, jealousy, and remorse.
One says: "The chief mental characteristic
of hysterical patients is an excessive
emotional excitability unchecked by
voluntary exertion." And again: "This
excessive emotional activity necessarily
induces exhaustion." The treatment of this
affection recognizes, first and last, the
influence of mind over body. We find that
moral suasion, the employment of the
individual in directions without herself, the
cultivation of an intellectual purpose, of an
objective quality of mind, are remedies that
rank with the nervines and antispasmodics in
the treatment of this disorder.

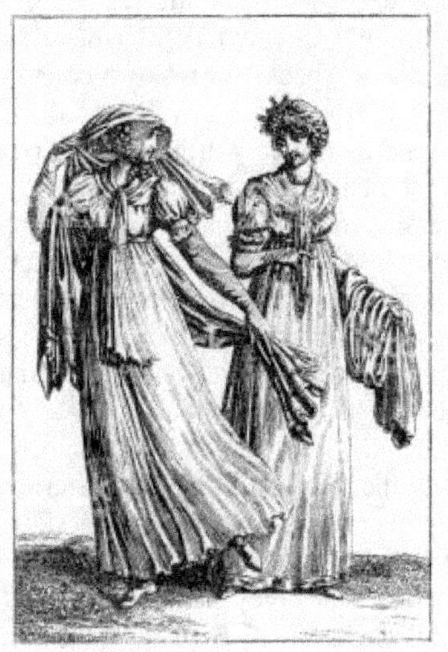

Modes de 1807. — 9, Costume pour la promenade.

As regards nervous exhaustion, Ave find
that affection is almost entirely confined to
the more highly civilized portions of the
community—indeed, is a disease of
civilization. Among the causes of nervous
exhaustion this same truth is manifest—that
excessive demands upon the individual
exciting the complex emotions of anxiety,
worry, are largely responsible for inducing
this affection. We believe, indeed, that hard
work, unaccompanied by emotional
excitement, seldom injures either man or
woman. It is the man who, in addition to
close application to work, is harrassed by
fears of poverty, of loss of position, of
anxieties for himself or his family, and the
woman who bears the burden of domestic
cares, of private griefs, or sustains the strain
of a complex social system, who suffers
from nervous exhaustion, not the bard-
working mechanic, or the unemotional
washer-woman. The experience of every
school-girl testifies that mental anxiety
produces a degree of physical exhaustion out
of all proportion to the muscular work
effected. The agitations of school politics,
the over-emotional character often infused
into school-girl friendships, the fears of
failure and kindred commotions result in
more physical weariness than hours of calm,
steady work in the laboratory or in the class-
room.

A college graduate confesses that one of the
most exhausting experiences of her college
life was a morning spent in absolute
physical inactivity in a student's meeting,
but in a state of mental commotion
impossible to describe, over an absorbing
issue in college politics. "After four hours of
that experience," she said, "I was fit for bed,

and for nothing else." It requires no great
ingenuity to suggest that this tendency in the
training of woman which affects her mental
and physical health, may be met by remedies
addressed to body and mind alike. The
education which shall discipline, not
eradicate, the emotional susceptibility of
women must begin where the gentility of Dr.
Holmes's ideal gentleman began, with our
great-grandmothers.

Heredity may not be able to shoulder all of
the sins of mankind, but, at least, it must
bear its share. The coming woman must not
only be well-born, she must be bred in more
hygienic methods. She must not only
possess inherited vigor, she must also be
educated nearer to Nature. The genuine
child of Nature is not a morbidly emotional
child. The girl who lives in the open air,
who knows every bird and flower and brook
in the neighborhood, has neither time nor
inclination to spend in reading the
sentimental histories of departed childsaints,
and takes small delight in morbid
conversation.

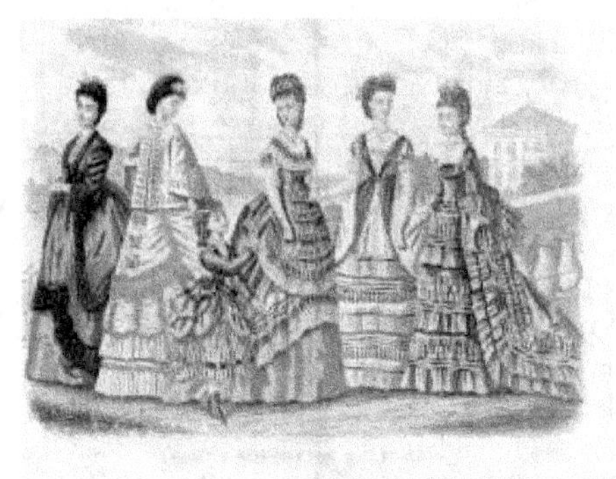

Out-of-door life has never been made popular or interesting for little girls as it always has been for boys. Girls will voluntarily seek fresh air and sunshine if they appreciate the delightful occupations as well as the *fun* to be found in it. They are quite right in "hating to go out because there is nothing to do." Open wide to them the fascinating book of Nature; let them read the story of bird-life and animal-life, and find their first hints of the wonders of plants and rocks by sunlight, and at first hand, not from a printed page in unventilated libraries. Then, when out-of-door life and out-of-door sports have been made as attractive and popular for girls as for boys, and when they have accepted the creed that a nobly-developed and active body is as much their birthright and glory as it has always been the glory of their brothers, we shall find we have gone a long way toward reducing exaggerated emotions in women. And if our first antidote for this condition lies in physical activity and in the cultivation of a sound body, the second antidote will be found in the provision of constant, congenial employment for the mind.

When a young woman went to Henry Ward Beecher to ask him to prescribe for her disappointed affections, he promptly advised her to begin the study of the higher mathematics! There is no doubt but that among the less apparent, but no less real causes of undue emotional development among women we may count the lack of congenial and effective work. There is nothing sanitary in intellectual idleness. Physiology forbids that the inactive brain should be a healthy one. The overworked individual may suffer from undue strain, but

the mind which is denied congenial
employment suffers even a worse penalty in
the disability of its best powers, and the
waste of purposeless energy.

Women who are receiving the so-called
higher education, find in its discipline and
opportunity the best remedy for any
tendency to excessive emotional
disturbance. "The worst enemy of the
emotions is the intellect." There is no
stronger argument for opening to women
new avenues for the acquisition of
knowledge than these facts of her
constitution offer, justified as the experiment
has been by those who have found life a
better and a broader thing to them because
of these opportunities.

Undoubtedly the actual erudition that is
gained in a collegiate training for women
could be obtained under other conditions
than in the four years of college life. But the
inestimable value of our women's colleges
lies not so much in their opportunities for
actual learning, as in the atmosphere they
offer. To live for four years under a *régime*
where mental and physical energy are
carefully utilized and disciplined, and where
the tendency is toward the development of
an objective type of mind and the cultivation
of a broad intellectual outlook—these are
incalculable benefits to woman.

Give to our children, our growing girls, and
our young women occupation which,
according to their age and capacity, shall
develop every faculty of the mind and afford
genuine scope for usefulness, and we shall
find that the energy which might have been
dissipated in unproductive emotions, has

been diverted into channels of effective work, and conserved for high and healthful ends.

THE most recent measurements of skeletons indicate that the ancients •were not superior to the moderns in stature, but may have been inferior. The average heights of two lots of Romano-British skeletons ranged from four feet ten inches for women to five feet two inches for the larger men; and the average height of twenty-five mummies in the British Museum is fifty-five inches for females and sixty-one inches for males.

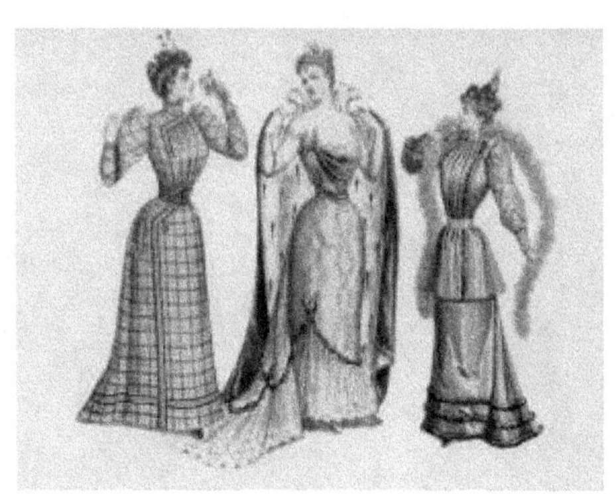

www.ingramcontent.com/pod-product-compliance
Lightning Source LLC
Chambersburg PA
CBHW061330250726
48657CB00003B/1106